THE DISTINCTIONS ON THE SOUL AND THE SPIRIT

THE DISTINCTIONS ON THE SOUL AND THE SPIRIT

CONSTANTINE THE AFRICAN

DALCASSIAN PRESS
Dark Age & Medieval Texts

Translator: Curtin, D.P. (1985-)

ISBN: 979-8-3495-2544-5 (Paperback)
ISBN: 979-8-3495-2545-2 (eBook)
Library of Congress Control Number:

Printed by Ingram Content Group, 1 Ingram Blvd, La Vergne, Tennessee
First Printing 2025, Dalcassian Press, Wilmington, DE

This work is part of a series produced in association with the Scriptorium Project and its community of scholars and translators.
Please visit our website at: www.thescriptoriumproject.com

THE DISTINCTIONS ON THE SOUL AND THE SPIRIT

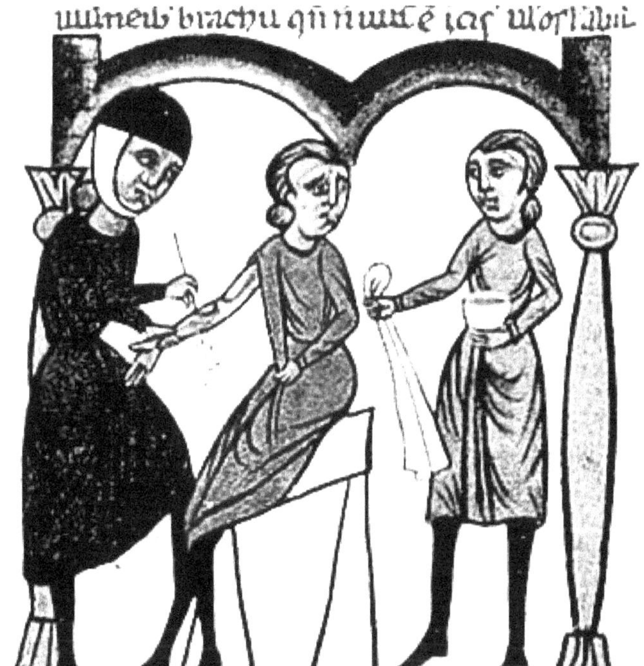

If one wishes to know the difference that exists between two things, it is necessary for him first to know what each of them is, because it is impossible to know the difference between two things unless he knows what each of them is; and thus, having understood the nature of each, he will be able to know the difference. And since we want to clarify the difference between the soul and the spirit, it is necessary to first speak about the soul and the spirit, and then about the difference that exists between the two. But as it is fitting for this work, let us begin with the spirit, and then follow with a discussion about the soul. The spirit is a certain subtle body that arises in the human body from the heart, and is carried in the pulsating veins to vivify the body, and it operates life and breathing, as well as pulse; similarly, it arises from the brain in the nerves, and operates sensation and motion. And some of the commendable physicians and philosophers who have used the work of surgery in the hearts of living beings have thought that there are two ventricles or cavities in the heart, one indeed on its right side, and the other on its left, and in the two ventricles blood and spirit are contained. But in the right ventricle there is more blood than spirit. In the left, however, there is more spirit than blood, and from the right ventricle two veins proceed, one of which leads to the lung, and through it is the breath of the heart: for the heart contracts and expands, and through its extension and contraction, the pulse of the whole body is formed; and therefore the pulse indicates the proper passions of the heart, both equal and unequal, and diverse, which occur due to various impediments of the same heart, which happens to it from itself, or from neighboring members. Therefore, when the heart is extended, it draws through the aforementioned vein from the lung a part of the air, which enters the lung through breathing, to cool the natural heat that is in it, so that it may be this nourishment or sustenance of the same spirit that is contained in its ventricles; and when the heart contracts, it sends through this vein to the lung whatever generates in it vaporous substances, and expels them from the ignited heat that is in it, and the lung expels them from the body, and this vein is called the pulse. The other vein, however, is called by the Arabs alabar, and this vein, at its origin in the heart, divides into two divisions, one of which ascends seeking the upper parts of the heart. And from it proceed branches from the chest all the way to the extremities of the head, through which life is given; this part of the body, seeking the lower parts of the body, descends to the extremities of the feet, and branches proceed from it through which the lower part of the human body is vivified, and the branches of both aforementioned parts, the veins which are dispersed throughout the rest of the body, are called furienet, and this is the cause of human life. The human body is closer, through that which it grants to each; the spirit that is in the ventricles of the heart is finished. And the indication by which it is proven that human life, which occurs through this spirit, is evident from the exit of this spirit at the hour of death, the movement indeed of the belly and the mouth, of the lips and the chest. In those, there is a kind of sobbing, and gasping, and a crowd calls all these in Arabic 'annaza', that is, the retreat or exit of the soul, and its exit from the body is through the very path by which the air enters it, which goes out from the ventricles of the heart to the lungs through the vein that we previously mentioned, which passes from the heart into the lung to draw in air, and extract the vapor of smoke, and expels from the lung through the tube or channel of the lung, that is, through the throat it passes to the mouth, and its exit from the mouth happens at the time of the movement of the mouth, when it indeed opens the mouth and can no longer close it, but it is now necessary to close it, due to the nullification of life, and the spirit after its exit from it. The cause by which this spirit exits from the body, and the cause of death, and the cause of the speed, or the quality of its exit, the lightness indeed of death, or its heaviness, and its appearance in some men, or its concealment in others, also the cause of sudden death, and other such matters are foreign to this book, because they are of greater inquiry, and require primary proofs, and probable arguments from many medical texts, whose exposition is lengthy and therefore we dismiss the mention of them. It is clear from what we have said that life exists through this spirit, which is in the ventricles of the heart, and that the pulse and the gasp are constituted to the desire of this same spirit to cool it through the air that enters from outside, and through the expulsion of vapor and smoke from it. Now it is evident that the spirit which is in the ventricles of the heart is the cause of life and the gasp and pulse here are of the vital spirit, whose origin is from the heart. The spirit, indeed, which proceeds from the brain and passes to the other limbs of the body is called the animal spirit. Its nourishment or sustenance is the spirit which is in the ventricles of the heart, because of the divisions of the pulse, which is called 'alabachar', which is sent from the heart to the upper parts. Of the body, when all the parts of the head have arrived and penetrated it, they are all joined together and combined, and they are interwoven according to the texture, and from the very substances woven together, a certain part extends under the brain, descending into the lower brain, suitable for receiving the animal spirit, conveying to it the spirit of life, which we have said is in the ventricles of the heart. The brain is divided into two divisions, one of which is anterior, which is also larger; the other is posterior, and in that anterior part are the ventricles, having an entrance to a common space, which is in the middle of the brain. In the posterior part, however, there is one ventricle making a passage to the aforementioned space, which is common to the ventricles that are in the anterior brain. Therefore, the subtle substance that cuts the net, which is under the brain to the interior of the brain, when it has reached certain ventricles that are in the anterior brain, leads to that vital spirit, which passing from there to another ventricle, becomes more subtle there, is purified, and is adapted to receive the vital essence. The soul is preserved, and this becomes for it a kind of digestion and conversion into a certain subtler and clearer spirit. Then it passes from the ventricles into the space, and from the space into the posterior ventricle of the brain, and through that passage which is the common space, which is in the middle of the brain at the back, and in this transition, that is, the entrance through which the spirit goes, a certain particle of the brain's substance is held, similar to a worm being raised and deposited along the way. When this particle has been raised, a hole is opened that is between the common space, which is joined to the ventricles, and the posterior ventricle of the brain. However, when it has been deposited, it is closed. Therefore, when the hole has been opened, the spirit passes from the anterior brain to the posterior, and this happens only if it is necessary to recall something that has been given to oblivion, at the time, namely, when there is thought about the past. But if the hole has not been opened, the spirit does not pass to the posterior brain, nor does the person remember, nor can they respond to those things about which they are questioned. That opening of the hole, which occurs through the raising of that body which is similar to a worm, is different in humans in terms of speed and slowness. For this happens in some more slowly, and therefore they have slow memories, and slow responses, thinking much before answering; and thus it happens that whoever wants to remember something, tilts their head very much, or turns it back while keeping their eyes still, so that this position or figure may assist in opening the aforementioned hole, and so that the body may be able to move slightly. For the intellect, imagination, or thought, foresight, or knowledge is made through the spirit that is in the ventricle, which is shared with those two ventricles that are in the anterior brain. Therefore, when a person has thought or foreseen something, it is necessary for the passage or hole that is in the common space, which is joined to those two ventricles that are in the anterior part of the head, and the ventricle that is in its posterior part, to be closed, so that the spirit, namely, which is in the common space, can make delays, so that it may be strengthened, and this becomes for it a kind of increase in strength, for thinking and understanding, as one becomes stronger in thought and understanding, foresight and knowledge. Therefore, it happens to one who thinks to lower the head to the ground and to look at it much, and to bend oneself as if writing some script, or describing some figures in it, so that this is as if a help to lay down that body, which we said is similar to a worm above the hole of that descent, which the spirit passes through to the posterior parts of the body. The spirit, however, which is in that space, that is, in the middle ventricle, is diverse in humans. For in some it is subtle and clear, and here it will be rational, thoughtful, a disposer, and of good knowledge. In others, however, it will be the opposite; it will be such as mad and irrational, light and foolish. From the anterior ventricle of the brain, pairs of nerves proceed, of which one pair, that is, divisions, coming from the anterior ventricles are joined to the eyes, and through this sight is made, and these among other nerves are concave. It is necessary that the spirit sent to it be much collected, sufficient and clear, and mixed with no other body. Another pair of nerves is joined to the covering of the eyes, that is, the eyelids. The third is joined to the tongue, and through this, sensation and taste are formed. The fourth is joined to the palate. The fifth is joined to the tympanum of the ear, and through this, the sense of hearing is formed. The sixth descends to the exterior, providing them with sensation, and a certain part returns to the unity, moving so that it may be gathered together. The seventh is joined to the tongue, through which it moves, and similarly, the spirit operates through the nerves, which transfers from the brain to these limbs. And as a sign of this, when some accident occurs, the spirit is obstructed in the passages of all the nerves, and the spirit itself is prevented from reaching the limb, and the function of that limb is nullified, as the whiteness that gathers in the eye, which when separated from the spirit that is in the nerve, affects the sight. And just as mixtures, that is, bad humors and vapors, which obstruct and separate between the spirit itself and the tympanum of the ear, or the instrument of smell, or the instrument of taste, or the instrument of touch: they operate either through deafness, or the destruction of taste, or touch, or smell. When the passages are opened, either through medicine, or the direction of nature in the struggling infirmity, the limb returns, and is made sound and equal. It also proceeds from the part of the brain, and descends through the mouth of the neck, into all the branches, which are the knots of the spine, and from it many pairs of nerves are directed between each branch, namely one pair passing to the haematid, which is a certain flesh joined to the veins, through which the movement of the limbs occurs. There will be through this movement of hands and feet, and of the whole body. The sign of this is that if at any time someone has suffered from these nerves, the function of that limb is nullified, and its movement is diminished, or weakened, or destroyed, and this happens according to the quantity of the impediment that has been suffered in the same nerves. For we see the hand against the Athenian and whole, and the cause of some impediment does not appear in it, and yet it feels nothing, nor is it moved, and when such infirmities have been cured, through some medicine they can be opened again through the branches of the brain, as are medicines that cleanse the branches of the limbs, and open the very closures. It returns to the same limbs, and the movements: if the infirmity does not transfer the measure of healing, and the limbs themselves have not been so weakened that they cannot sustain healing, and perhaps it happens to the spirit, which is in all the ventricles, or in any of them, some impediment arises from a bad mixture, or from the combination of harmful vapors, and through this the action of the same member is destroyed. For example: when the spirit that is in the anterior ventricles has suffered some impediment or corruption, thus from this destruction of sensation occurs, just as happens to one who enters a bath and there makes delays. For his eyes are obscured, and he sees nothing. Or just as it happens to one in whom red bile is stirred up, and its vapor ascends to the head. If there is an impediment in the anterior part of the brain, the spirit that is in it is obscured, and it does not perceive anything, similarly affecting hearing and the other senses. For example, if there is an obstruction in the middle part of the brain, while the other parts remain intact, thought and cognition are destroyed, and only the senses and motion will remain equal. This is similar to what happens in melancholic illness, which is a mixture or disturbance of reason and destruction of cognition. If there is an obstruction in the upper or lower part of the brain, only memory is destroyed, while the other functions of man remain equal, that is, proper. However, if there is an obstruction in two of these ventricles, or in three, and it occupies the whole brain, there will be an impediment in cognition, sensation, and motion universally, like what happens in apoplexy and similar conditions. Therefore, it is conclusively proven that the spirit in the anterior ventricles operates sensation, that is, sight, hearing, taste, smell, and touch: and with these, it operates imagination, which the Greeks call phantasia, and the spirit in the middle ventricle operates thought, cognition, providence, memory, and motion. It is thus established from all these that there are two kinds of spirits in the human body: one, which is called vital, whose nourishment or sustenance is air, and its animation comes from the heart, and it is sent through the pulse to the rest of the body, and it operates life, pulse, and breathing. There is also another, which is called animal, which operates in the very brain, whose nourishment is vital spirit, and its emanation comes from the brain, and it operates in the brain thought and memory, and providence, and from it, it is sent through the nerves to the other members, to operate sensation and motion. To narrate something about the soul is indeed very grave and difficult, and this is evidenced by the diversity or discord of the principal philosophers, namely Plato and Aristotle, as well as those who came after them. But we will follow the definitions by which Aristotle and Plato defined it. In the definition and exposition of the soul, we utilize credible arguments, and this narrative follows the virtues of the soul, because it is sufficient to elucidate our intention at this point, namely the distinction between spirit and soul. Let us then say how the philosopher Plato defines the soul: he says, "The soul is an incorporeal substance that moves the body." Aristotle, however, in his definition of the soul says: "The soul is the perfection of a living and acting body, potentially." Now let us explain these two definitions, starting with the first, which is Plato's. We shall show that the soul is substance, and thus we say: Because whatever receives opposites, while being one in number and unchangeable in its essence, is substance. But the soul receives virtues and vices, while being one in number: Thus the soul of Plato, which is unchangeable in its essence, receives virtues and vices, which are opposites: Therefore, the soul receives opposites, while being one in number and unchangeable in its essence, thus it is substance. And let us say again: Whatever moves substance, is substance. But the soul moves the body, and the body is substance. And because it is already evident from clear arguments that the soul is substance, let us now show that the soul is incorporeal substance, and let us say. The qualities of every body are perceptible, and those qualities which are not perceived by corporeal sense are incorporeal. Therefore, the soul is incorporeal. Again: Every body is subject to all senses, or to some of them. But the soul is not subject to all senses, nor to any of them; therefore, the soul is not a body. Furthermore: Every body is either animated or inanimate; and if the soul is a body, it is either animated or inanimate. But it is impossible for it to be inanimate if it is a body, because it is inconsistent for it to be both soul and inanimate. And if we say that the soul is an animated body, it will be reiterated to us whether the soul is a body or not, and this will lead to infinity. Therefore, the soul is not a body. And again: If the soul is a subtle body, it will either be air or a subtle spirit, diffused throughout the whole body, or it will be fire; and if it is so, it is necessary that that spirit or fire has a proper species or proper virtue, because unless it has some proper species or proper virtue, that is, unless it has some property which fire or air does not have, it will be entirely air or fire of the soul. But if it has a proper species, that species will be the soul. Likewise: If the soul is a body, it is necessary that it be either a composite body or a simple one. If it is a simple body, it will undoubtedly be fire, or air, or earth, or water. And if the soul is one of these elements absolutely, that is, without a proper species by which it is distinguished from that which participates in its genus, because it is of the same genus, it will be the soul. Thus it is proven that if the soul is fire, it will be fire of the soul. And similarly about the other elements. And if it is so, every body that contains an element will be animated. For example: If it is air, the lung and the puff will be inflated and will be animated; and if the soul is water, it will be a full body animated with water, and such words are base and empty. Therefore, if the soul is a composed body, then it will be a body of the soul, and not a body. And because it is now clear that the soul becomes an incorporeal substance, let us now explain in what ways it moves the body, and let us say. That everything that is moved or moves by the motion of its mover, just as a plow is moved by the motion of oxen, or it is moved when that which moves it is not moved, because that which moves something either moves and moves, or does not; and this occurs in four ways. Because it will either be by its desire from which it is moved, just as it is moved by a beloved, towards that which it loves, or by hatred, or by flight, or by fear, just as an enemy is moved by his enemy, or against him: or by natural action, just as a stone is moved by weight, when the weight itself is immobile, or because that which moves is the principal cause, or the cause of that which is moved, just as mastery is the cause of the motion of the master and that mastery is not moved by the motion of the master. Thus, the soul moves the body, and it is not moved by its motion. Therefore, the soul is the cause of the motion of animals, through will and action, and change, and it is not moved in any way by the change of the body, since it is incorporeal. Let us see, therefore, from these modes we have mentioned, in what manner the soul moves the body. Let us say that the soul moves the body in a fourth way from a fruitful species of motion, namely, it moves the body while it itself is immobile. It also moves because it is the principal occasion, or the cause of its motion, because man acts through it, that is, through the soul. And just as mastery is the cause of the motion of the master, and that mastery is not moved by the motion of the master, so the soul moves the body, but is not moved by its motion. Therefore, the soul is the cause of the motion of animals, through desire and will, and through action and change, and it is not moved in any way by the modes of the motion of the body, since it is incorporeal. And since we have now exposed the definition of Plato in which he defined the soul, and have revealed the interpretation of all its parts: now let us discuss the definition of Aristotle the philosopher. Aristotle, indeed the prince of philosophers, defined the soul as follows. For he said that it is the perfection of the acting and living body potentially. In his book that he wrote about the soul, he gave such a definition of the soul, saying: The soul is the perfection of a natural living instrument potentially. He said potentially because certain things are said to be potential, and certain things by effect. When through the generic things it is designated by effect, perfection is indeed the reception of its species. For this reason, he says the soul is perfection, because something is animated potentially, and when it has been animated by effect, then it is said to be perfect, and its perfection is the reception of its species, that is, to be animated, sensible, and voluntarily movable. It is established, therefore, what we have said, that the soul is the species of the animal without doubt, and since it is the perfection of the same animal. For the perfection of a thing is the reception of its species, and since it is truly proven that the soul is a species, and we call this species perfection, it is necessary for us to enumerate the modes of perfection and to choose which of them pertains to the soul. Therefore, let us say that perfection is spoken of in two ways. There is indeed a first perfection and a second. The first perfection in man is the second perfection in man studying; in those things which he knows through sciences and masteries. For example, a physician is called the first perfection due to the knowledge of medicine. When he begins to operate on what he knows, he is called the second perfection. Therefore, the soul is the first perfection because one who sleeps, and if he lacks sense, during the time of sleep, he still has a sensible soul, and every species, and perfection, is the species and perfection of some thing. Therefore, the soul is the species atop the perfection of the body. There are two modes of bodies, for there are certain bodies in which the natural species of animals, trees, fire, and water exist, and whatever has natural motion within itself. There are certain qualities by which a species is acquired through mastery, such as office and deceit. Therefore, the soul is the species of a natural body, because the body does not arise from the acts of mastery. The natural species differs from the species of mastery, because the natural species is substance, and the species of mastery is an accident. Therefore, the soul is substance, because it is the species of a natural body. The modes of natural bodies are two, because some are composite, while others are simple. Simple ones are, for example, air, fire, water, earth. Composite ones are, for example, animals, trees. However, the soul is not the species of a simple body, but of a composite natural one, because whatever has a soul is animated, that is, it lives, and whatever lives is convertible or dissoluble, and it necessarily requires food, by which it can recover what has been dissolved from it, and which aids its vegetation by giving it growth. Food requires various instruments, some of which are necessary for it to be carried to the body to restore it, to run, and to penetrate, such as the throat, veins in animals, and the trunk of the tree in trees, and some are necessary for the restored body, to expel from it what is superfluous, such as pores in animals, or exits, and vessels in trees. Instruments also multiply in animals due to their size, perfection, and the multitude of their functions. If it is an animal, it has members of life, such as the heart, brain, and whatever is joined to them. What becomes sensible will be the nerves and senses. If, however, it is mobile, it will voluntarily be the nerves and flesh, and if it is so, it is well and rightly said that the soul is the first perfection of the living natural body instrumentally. And this definition is universal, abundant, and sufficient for every soul that has been in a corruptible or dissoluble body universally. However, it seems to corrupt the first particle and place in its stead a living being potentially; it does not greatly differ from an animal, because the interpretation of both definitions is one. For when it says "living potentially," it intended to convey that the body was thus in its essence before it became a soul, or prior to receiving the soul, which could potentially live. But it wanted to be understood through what it said about "living potentially," that it was an instrument capable of being used for acts of life. Therefore, it signifies instrumental, which is living potentially. This is the definition Aristotle provided, along with its exposition that we have set forth, and we have revealed each part of it. And because we have already exposed their definitions, namely those of Plato and Aristotle, and we have disclosed the interpretation of each part of them, let us now speak about the virtues of the soul and say that the primary virtues of the soul, which are its material in strength, as if they were kinds, are three: the first is the vegetative, the second, the sensitive, and the third, the rational. And these virtues are called according to the disposition of the soul. For the soul is said to be sensitive, and the vegetative soul is beastly and mobile, which moves voluntarily; and the rational soul uses reason, cognition, & thought. The vegetative soul, which in other books is called the soul of plants, is common to us with trees, herbs, and animals. And the sensitive soul, which is elsewhere called the vital soul, is common to us with animals. The rational soul, on the other hand, is proper to man. The function of the vegetative soul is to nourish and grow, and it does this through four powers called natural. These are attractive, retentive, digestive, and expulsive; and this function is found in all vegetation, that is, in trees, herbs, and also in animals, and in man. The functions of the sensitive soul, which is called vital, are seven: namely, vision, hearing, taste, smell, and touch, which are the five senses of the body, and imagination, and voluntary motion from place to place; and these functions are found in all animate beings, that is, in animals and man. The functions of the rational soul are knowledge, foresight, estimation, doubt, understanding, and memory; and these functions are proper to man among other animals. Since with God's help we have now explained what spirit and soul are, let us now speak of the difference that exists between them. Let us say that the first difference is this: namely, that spirit is corporeal. The soul, however, is incorporeal. And that the spirit is comprehended by the body, but the soul is not. And when the spirit is separated from the body, it perishes. However, the functions of the soul, when separated from the body, perish, but the soul itself does not perish in itself. The soul, moreover, when it is in the body, moves the body and provides it with sensation and life through the mediator spirit; and the spirit operates this without any mediator. The soul moves the body and provides it with life because it is the primary cause of this, and it operates in it. The spirit, which operates this, is the secondary cause. Therefore, the spirit is the cause of the life of the body and its sensation, and motion, and the other actions of it are more immediate, while the soul is the cause of this in a more extended sense. For when the human body is composed of very diverse parts, which are hard and soft, such as flesh and bone, nerves as well as tendons, and other similar things; and of moist parts, which are humors, namely blood and phlegm, and both choleras, and of the spirit which is in the ventricles of the heart, and in the brain, in the pulse as well in the nerves: every spirit that is more subtle and clearer in these parts will be more capable of receiving the actions of the soul and more suitable for the other parts of the body, and according to the quality of its subtlety and clarity, it will receive from the actions of the soul. For this reason, the philosophers said that the virtues of the soul follow the compositions of the body. Therefore, whose composition of the body is in perfection and qualities, his spirit that is in his body will be in perfection of equality, and the actions of the soul will be similarly so. However, whose composition of the members has been in its proper temperament and is less perfect, the spirit will be imperfect in what is owed from subtlety, and the actions of the soul will be more imperfect for this reason. And thus, the virtues of the soul are imperfect in children and weaker in women, and similarly in nations whose composition is weaker because of heat or cold, due to their proximity to the soul, affects the length of the veins. There are Ethiopians, Slavs, and those similar to them. Because of this, the actions of the soul in the spirit are diverse, and since they occur through the spirit, they are questioned in the heart, life, breath, and pulse, solely because the spirit itself is closer to the air than the other spirits and is less subtle. Then, through the spirit that is in the anterior ventricles of the brain, there are sensations and thoughts, because it has acquired an increase in subtlety above the spirit that is in the heart. Then, through the spirit that is in the subsequent ventricles, there is thought and foresight, due to the fact that it has received from the subtlety above another spirit, and because it is necessary for it to have an abundance of subtlety when it wishes to remember something, whether it has passed or its time has been prolonged. Therefore, these things about the differences between spirit and soul should suffice for you.

The book on the difference between soul and spirit ends here.

This work was produced in association with:

THE SCRIPTORIUM PROJECT

DALCASSIAN PRESS

Dark Age & Medieval Texts

Wilmington, DE

www.ingramcontent.com/pod-product-compliance
Lightning Source LLC
LaVergne TN
LVHW050940210926
848482LV00013B/685
9798349525445